This Journal Belongs to:

.........................................................................................................................

# GENDER IDENTITY JOURNAL

## Prompts and Practices for Exploration and Self-Discovery

**Katie Leikam,** MBA, LCSW

ROCKRIDGE
PRESS

Interior and Cover Designer: Linda Kocur
Art Producer: Hannah Dickerson
Editor: Nora Spiegel
Production Editor: Matthew Burnett
Production Manager: Riley Hoffman

Cover art used under license from Shutterstock.com
Author photograph courtesy of Bonnie Heath.

Paperback ISBN: 978-1-63807-708-4
R0

# CONTENTS

# INTRODUCTION

Welcome to the *Gender Identity Journal*. Exploring your gender identity can be an emotional, sensitive journey in your life, one that is filled with questions and self-reflection about the core of who you are as a person. Whether you are just starting to have feelings and questions about your gender identity, are in the middle of your exploration, or are already certain what your gender identity is, this journal will help you get to know yourself even better and discover what gender identity makes you feel most comfortable in your own life.

I am a licensed clinical social worker who is a therapist, gender specialist, and a GEI-certified member of the World Professional Association for Transgender Health (WPATH). Over the years, I have worked with hundreds of transgender, genderqueer, and nonbinary clients, including both teenagers and adults, to help them explore their gender identities and, if they decide they want to, start living publicly as their authentic or affirmed selves. I started this work because a great friend transitioned over a decade ago, and I wanted to break down the barriers that the transgender community faced with professionals at the time.

This journal will guide you through the self-reflection that's important when you are first exploring your gender identity, or anytime during your own unique transition and affirmation process. Before you get started on your reflection, it is important to go over some relevant terms about gender identity. You may be aware of these terms already, but a refresher can be helpful.

## How to Use This Journal

This is *your* journal. Since it is only yours, it is a safe space for you to explore your gender identity without worrying about the opinions of others. This is a place where you can reflect on your past and your present in your own words. While sometimes the prompts and exercises can be challenging and bring up difficult emotions, you get to set the pace of your exploration. If it gets overwhelming, set it aside for a bit. The hope is that with the use of this journal, you will gain a better understanding of your gender identity. You can use this journal on your own, or, if you are working with a therapist, you can share excerpts in session with them.

There is no shame in seeking support from a therapist, support group, or psychiatrist if you find yourself experiencing anxiety, depression, or some other emotional concern during your gender exploration. Keep in mind that this book does not replace professional help. If you ever experience feelings of being a danger to yourself, please seek professional help or call emergency services. You can also find helpful resources in the Resources appendix (page 148).

This book is divided into sections based on where you might be in your gender exploration. Each section has prompts and exercises to start your thinking and help you work through your feelings. You don't have to use this book from start to finish; you can flip back and forth throughout. If you are just starting out, you may want to begin in section 1. If you are ready to come out or tell people your gender identity, section 4 might be a good place to start.

## A Brief Primer on Gender Identity

You and I may have grown up thinking that gender was binary, only male and female, but gender is far more complex than that. I am about to tell you about many different gender identities that may be unfamiliar to you, very familiar to you, or somewhere in between. These terms give voice to the complex experience and possibilities of gender identity and will help you gain deeper insight as you explore your own gender identity.

*Gender identity* is the gender that you personally know yourself to be and how you choose to express it. *Gender* is based on societal expectations around various behaviors and characteristics, including legal and social statuses. Your *gender role* is the way that you were told to relate to others out in the world based on those societal norms; however, trans and nonbinary people may have never related to or adhered to these norms. When you were born, a doctor looked at your genitals and assigned you a *sex* based on what they perceived your biological characteristics to be. This *assigned sex* might not match your gender identity. (The term *biological sex* is never an okay term to use; it is inaccurate, is often used by anti-trans activists to diminish a person's lived experience of gender, and is considered hurtful. It is best, if absolutely necessary, to say *assigned sex at birth* or *assigned gender*.)

Your gender identity might not fit into society's binary expectations around gender, and as you grow up, your sense of yourself and your identity will continue to evolve. Your *gender expression* is the way you present yourself to others, and it does not have to match your assigned sex. When people talk about *presenting* as a certain gender, they generally mean that a person is outwardly expressing themself in a way that fits within the gendered role for a certain gender.

Though our world is saturated with messaging that gender is binary (e.g., public restrooms, clothing departments, etc.), gender identity is far from binary. When you look at identity in terms of feminine and masculine and all identities in between and outside of them, you will see that gender exists on a *spectrum*. Some people feel both male and female at the same time, or an identity outside of the constraints of binary gender. Some people are *agender*, meaning they feel like they don't have a gender, or like they have a neutral gender.

Someone who is *transgender* has a gender identity that is different than the sex they were assigned at birth. When someone is transgender and they are going through the process of changing how the world sees them and refers to them, and affirming themself through this process, it is said that they are *transitioning*. People can transition socially, medically, or both. When people socially transition, they may change their outward appearance through different hairstyles or clothing, and they may ask people to use a different name and pronouns for them. When people medically transition, they might change their body shape and appearance using hormonal medications or through gender-affirming surgery. However, it's important to keep in mind that transitioning and coming out are unique for everyone and can take many different forms based on your personal journey. Not everyone who is transgender will socially or medically transition, and that does not make them any less valid in their gender identity.

It's important to note that if you are transgender, your assigned gender does not have any bearing on your *sexual orientation*. Someone can be transgender and be attracted to people of a different gender identity. Likewise, someone can be transgender and be attracted to someone of the same gender identity or multiple gender identities.

## Different Gender Identities and Terminology

There is no single authority on gender identity or the labels that describe gender identity, but there are common identities that many people connect with. Gender identity is personal, and no one can tell you who you are. Your identity is yours to claim. It can be useful to review some of the different gender identity terms people use, as many people find it empowering to name this aspect of themselves. You will see that some of these identities overlap with one another. That is because gender exists on a spectrum, and some identities fall within the same area of the spectrum.

**Agender**  People who are agender typically identify as having no gender at all, or identify with neither binary gender.

**Binary**  Binary refers to the classification of people as either male or female, whether in regard to sex or gender. This may include how society expects a person to present themself outwardly, or a person's perceived biological characteristics. Referring to someone only according to binary terms is offensive because it marginalizes people who have other gender identities on the spectrum.

**Cisgender**  People who feel that their gender aligns with the sex they were assigned at birth.

**Demiboy**  Demiboy is a nonbinary gender and describes someone who somewhat identifies as masculine, but not fully. (One does not have to be transmasculine [see page xii] to identify as a demiboy.)

**Demigirl** Demigirl is a nonbinary gender and describes someone who somewhat feels more feminine but does not fully identity as a woman. (One does not have to be transfeminine [see page xii] to identify as a demigirl.)

**Genderfluid** Genderfluid people experience changing feelings of being both masculine and feminine (or somewhere else on the spectrum) for short and prolonged periods of time.

**Genderqueer** Genderqueer people feel like they do not fit in a societally typical male or female role or gender identity. Genderqueer can be a term that is used when someone rejects the societal labels of male and female. A similar term is **gender nonconforming**, which refers to someone with a gender expression (but not always a gender identity) that differs from the norm.

**Gender dysphoria** This is not an identity, but is the internal sense of discomfort caused by one's gender not aligning with their physical self or the gender they were assigned at birth. Often, steps like social or medical transition are taken to alleviate this discomfort. Gender dysphoria is also the definition and diagnosis used by physicians and other medical professionals to treat trans, gender-nonconforming, and nonbinary patients/clients. That said, this has often been reduced to a very limiting notion of what it could mean to be trans, and one doesn't need to have dysphoria to be valid or to feel a need to transition.

**Identified gender** This is the internal feeling someone has of their gender. In recent times, most people have stopped using this term—one does not identify (or choose) their gender, they are just the gender they are. A term that may be more suitable is *affirmed gender*.

**Intersex** A person who is intersex is born with variations in sex characteristics that do not fall cleanly one one side of the male/female binary, and those variations can include hormonal, internal, or external physical characteristics. Being intersex does not necessarily mean someone is transgender.

**Nonbinary** This is a term that encompasses gender identities that are not rooted in the binary of male and female or masculine and feminine.

# Keep in Mind

There are a few vital pieces of information to know before you begin exploring your gender identity. These are valuable tips to keep in mind throughout your journey and while you are processing feelings related to your gender identity.

- Your gender identity is your own and no one can take your gender identity away from you.

- You are the authority on your own gender identity.

- Even if you are not presenting outwardly as your gender identity, you still are your gender identity.

- Your path of self-discovery toward your gender identity can take weeks, years, or an entire lifetime, and some people have a slower exploration. For other people, their gender identity seems to just click in their head one day. Neither way is right or wrong.

- Remember that the process of discovering your gender identity can be joyful, or it can bring up difficult emotions—and often both. Don't get so caught up in the challenging aspects that you forget you are discovering your authentic self—that in itself is deeply meaningful!

- This exploration is about you. It's not about what your family, friends, or partner(s) might think about your identity.

- In the beginning, let go of the categories that people put gender identity into. Allow yourself the space and freedom to explore the feelings inside yourself without needing to attach a label to them right away.

- The goal of this journal is not to find a label, it's to know yourself authentically and on your own terms. Your gender identity does not have to fit into a box or match a label that society has created.

**Transfeminine** This is a term used by people who were assigned male at birth, but who typically identify as feminine and may present more feminine.

**Transgender/trans** Someone who does not identify with the sex they were assigned at birth or the gender that society expects them to be.

**Transmasculine** This is a term used by people who were assigned female at birth, but who typically identify as masculine and may present more masculine.

**Two Spirit** This is a term that is used by Indigenous North Americans and refers to people outside of the gender binary within Indigenous communities past and present. Two Spirit people often hold important societal and ceremonial roles. (Keep in mind that use of this term by people who aren't of Indigenous lineage is considered appropriative and offensive.)

## What Does Gender Exploration Look Like?

Gender exploration can be exciting, but it can also bring to the surface emotions such as fear, hesitation, and shame, and it can put pressure on the relationships you have with people around you. There are many challenges people face when they embark on exploring their gender identity. These can be challenges within themselves, such as fighting the societal norms that have been embedded within all of us. There can be challenges with society and people they know, such as misunderstanding, rejection, prejudice, and sometimes hostility, and they may need to learn how to stand up to adversity. I have seen people experience overwhelming joy when they discover their gender identity and take steps to affirm and express that identity. It is a beautiful thing to witness people embracing and honoring their affirmed self, sometimes after years of suppressing their feelings. Even in the face of adversity, knowing who you truly are can be empowering. Each person's path and circumstances are different, and empowerment will look very different for everyone.

There is a difference between exploring your gender and transitioning. Exploring your gender is undergoing an internal self-reflection, where transitioning refers to the process of embracing one's self in an affirmed gender; it very often refers to making changes to your physical being or physical presentation to address gender dysphoria, whether it is by taking hormonal therapy, living publicly in your affirmed gender, or pursuing any other medical and social steps that affirm your sense of self. You don't have to socially or medically transition during or after your gender identity exploration, but some people find that is the best way to live their lives fully, in any gender identity. Some people will find they have no desire to physically transition at all, or they might discover that they are cisgender and enjoy experimenting with different forms of gender expression. This journal is primarily intended for people who are exploring their gender, but people who have already transitioned can find value in this self-exploration as well.

People who explore their gender identity and find that they are not cisgender may want to come out or disclose this information to others, whether privately or publicly. You may ask people to call you by a different name or use different pronouns. For most people, coming out is not a one-time event, but a lifelong, selective process as they navigate new relationships and social situations.

You have taken a big step by picking up this journal and deciding that you are ready to explore your gender identity. Wherever your exploration may lead, try to keep an open mind and enjoy the journey. Remember to be gentle with yourself and to take breaks when you need. Now, let's get started!

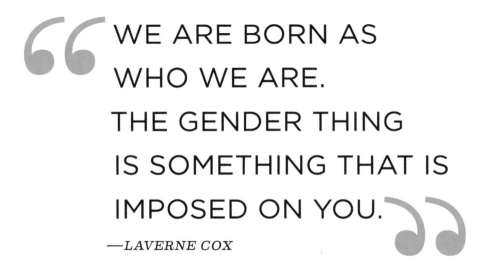

**"WE ARE BORN AS WHO WE ARE. THE GENDER THING IS SOMETHING THAT IS IMPOSED ON YOU."**

—*LAVERNE COX*

# 1

# Laying the Groundwork
# for Your Exploration

Going on any journey requires preparation. This section of your journal will inspire you to lay the groundwork as you explore your gender identity. You'll delve into why this is important and what led you to start thinking about your gender identity in the first place. The prompts and exercises will help you gauge where you are with your gender identity, explore the fears and obstacles in your way, and challenge you to dig deep in your process of self-exploration.

# Gender Identity Self-Assessment Check-In

*Please answer each question true or false.*

1   I wish I saw someone of a different gender when I look in the mirror. **T / F**

2   Going into a restroom for the gender I was assigned at birth doesn't bother me, and I sometimes prefer it. **T / F**

3   I don't really care about the gender role expectations of my assigned gender, such as men being powerful or women being nurturing. **T / F**

4   There have been times I wished I could be a different gender. **T / F**

5   Sometimes I have difficulty during intimacy because of certain aspects of my physical self, or I disassociate during sex to get out of my body. **T / F**

6   I like to shop in the clothing section that is expected for someone of my designated sex. **T / F**

7   I watch transition videos on YouTube or TikTok or follow transgender people on Instagram because I am interested in transition stories. **T / F**

8   I find pleasure with my partners when intimate, and feel proud and comfortable with the way my body is while we are enjoying one another. **T / F**

**9** When puberty began, although I may have been nervous, I had an easy time accepting the ways in which my body was changing.  **T / F**

**10** I don't think about changing my gender presentation. I feel content with my gender presentation.  **T / F**

**11** There are things I would like to change about my hairstyle, how I dress, or my voice, because those things are currently uncomfortable to me.  **T / F**

**12** I feel uncomfortable when people make gender-related assumptions about me based on my assigned gender.  **T / F**

### Self-Assessment:

■ If your answers to questions 1, 4, 5, 7, 11, and 12 were mostly true, you may want to begin exploring your gender identity to think about the uneasy feelings you have about your assigned gender.

■ If your answers to questions 2, 3, 6, 8, 9, and 10 were mostly true, you may be secure in your assigned gender or you may want to explore alternate ways to express yourself.

It's always important at the start of any journey to know why you are going on it in the first place. Knowing the *why* can help you when times get tough and when you may want to stop or take a pause. So, why did you pick up this journal? What do you hope to gain from exploring your gender identity? Is it peace, comfort, resolution, or another feeling you seek? Write about and reflect on the feelings you desire.

Many of my clients have told me there was a meme they looked at, a television show they watched, or something someone said that made them immediately question their gender, and that this came as a surprise to them. Was there a "click" that your gender may be different than how you have been expressing it? Was there a moment or situation that pushed you to begin to question your gender?

There may have been times in your life when you wondered what would happen if you were a different gender than the one you were assigned. These thoughts might have come during times of deep introspection, or they could have been more playful thoughts that were just passing through your mind. Have you thought about yourself as any gender besides your assigned gender before? Reflect on how you saw yourself when you had these thoughts.

# What Does Your Wardrobe Hold?

For this exercise, go to your closet and look at the articles of clothing in it. Is the majority of your clothing traditionally designed for one gender? What feelings do your clothes elicit? When you look at your closet full of clothes, think about if what you see actually portrays how you feel about your gender identity. Do you feel affirmed when you look at the clothes you wear every day, or do you feel like you could use a change?

You may have heard the term *gender dysphoria* before reading this journal. This term is generally used in two ways. The first is as a diagnosis used by providers of medical and mental health care. The second is a way of describing the incongruence, discomfort, or distress one might feel when they think about their assigned gender, the state of their body, their gender presentation, or how people perceive their gender. Does this term resonate with your experience? What do you feel when you hear the phrase gender dysphoria? Are these feelings strong, neutral, or weak? If your feelings are intense, ask yourself what it is about gender dysphoria that is bringing those feelings up.

It is common to experience shame or discomfort surrounding gender questioning or gender dysphoria, and it may come and go, or feel more or less intense at times or during certain activities. It's important to know that you don't have to have negative feelings of dysphoria to be transgender, but some people do experience them. What is happening in your life when your questioning or dysphoria intensifies? Are you in public or private? Are you just thinking, or are you gazing at your reflection? Are you in a relationship with someone else? Think about where, when, and why you experience these feelings.

Gender questioning or dysphoria can lead to you feeling uncomfortable in social situations, because you may not be presenting to the world as your actual gender identity. These feelings can sometimes make people stay home more often, or they can find it hard to be in front of a lot of people. Reflect on whether gender questioning or dysphoria has prevented you from doing something you wanted or needed to do.

# Build a Toolbox Full of Coping Skills

Imagine you are a mechanic, and you are working on fixing a car. You come to work with a toolbox full of tools. Just as a mechanic carries around a toolbox of tools, you can carry around a toolbox of coping skills. Coping skills are tools you use to fix yourself when you are broken down like the car. Examples of helpful coping skills are deep breathing, talking to a trusted friend, or various self-care activities. Imagine you are the mechanic carrying a toolbox of coping skills. Draw your toolbox and fill it in with your coping skills.

Sometimes emotions can be a stumbling block to self-reflection. Those pesky emotions that bring us down, like sadness or fear of isolation, can block our ability to think through our other emotions fully. Getting to a place of self-reflection means that sometimes you have to look those emotions in the eye and say "Not now." Do you have any strong or negative internal emotions blocking you from thinking about gender identity?

When we have these passing thoughts, or when we are in deep reflection, we can have a flood of emotions in the moment. Sometimes that flood of emotions can be negative, positive, or both at the same time. In times when you have thought of yourself as another gender identity, did these thoughts have negative or positive—or a combination of both—connotations for you?

How we grew up and the lessons we were taught about our identities and gender norms can stay with us for our entire lives. Sometimes we have to go through a process of breaking the norms we were taught as a child. Do you have any internal obstacles keeping you from exploring your gender identity, such as the way your family talked to you about gender roles when you were growing up?

# Conquering Your Obstacle Wall

Sometimes, when things get hard, we forget how strong we are. You might be stuck in your exploration because you have hit a wall of shame. Remember to be kind and gentle to yourself and take a break if it is needed. But if you are ready, take a moment to look back on your life and think of the last three times you were faced with a wall of doubt and shame. How did you climb over the wall those previous times? Write those down.

Consider what has changed since the last wall you climbed over. What strategies would you use now to climb over an obstacle wall? Find a blank sheet of paper and list out as many as you can think of. Keep this list in your wallet or billfold so that you have a physical reminder of strategies to help you overcome challenges you may face in the future.

There are lots of things that keep people from exploring their gender identity. You might be thinking, "What would my boss or coworkers think? How would I ever talk to my family?" Do you have any external obstacles keeping you from exploring your gender identity, such as work, a relationship, or your family? Can you write about these obstacles?

Exploring your gender identity may elicit some uncomfortable feelings, and it can be tough to experience these. Some of the feelings you uncover may feel new or different, or you may be apprehensive about experiencing them. Are there things you fear about the possibility that your gender identity is different than your assigned gender? What is it about these things that you are afraid of? (Please remember: If at any time you are feeling like this is too much, be kind to yourself and take a break.)

# The Meditative Bowl Exercise

For this meditative exercise, grab a bowl of some sort and then sit somewhere comfortable with the bowl in front of you.

1. Close your eyes and gently and slowly run your finger around the rim of the bowl.

2. As you run your finger in the circle, start to breathe in and out, slowly and from your stomach. You can take your whole time running your finger around the rim for one breath in, and then again for one breath out.

3. As you breathe, try to focus your attention only on your breath and your finger moving around the rim of the bowl. Gently let go of any thoughts that pop up and refocus your attention on your breath and the bowl.

Follow this breathing pattern at least eight times and return to it whenever you need to reset, relax, or ground yourself.

"THESE YEARS IN SILENCE
AND REFLECTION MADE ME
STRONGER AND REMINDED
ME THAT ACCEPTANCE HAS
TO COME FROM WITHIN AND
THAT THIS KIND OF TRUTH
GIVES ME THE POWER TO
CONQUER EMOTIONS I DIDN'T
EVEN KNOW EXISTED."

—RICKY MARTIN

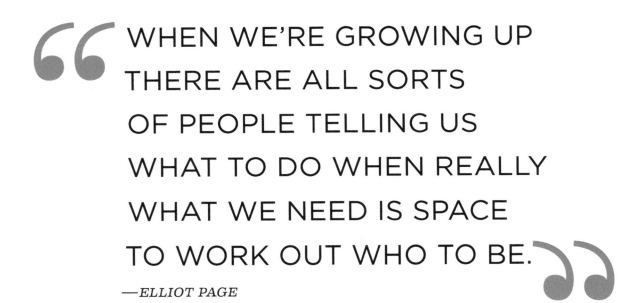

"WHEN WE'RE GROWING UP
THERE ARE ALL SORTS
OF PEOPLE TELLING US
WHAT TO DO WHEN REALLY
WHAT WE NEED IS SPACE
TO WORK OUT WHO TO BE."

—ELLIOT PAGE

# 2

# Reflecting on Who You've Been

An especially important part of gender identity exploration is reflecting on your past and how the construct of gender was imparted to you. In this section of the journal, you will identify the influences of prescribed gender roles in your childhood and adolescence, reflect on how you previously expressed your gender identity, investigate how you felt during puberty and name any gender discomfort you may have had, and start to break down gender stereotypes.

Our gender identity can be constructed from the messages we receive from the important people in our lives and the expectations they have for us. As a child, did your parents or guardians place any gendered expectations on you, such as the extracurricular activities you could participate or not participate in, the toys you could play with, or the clothes you could wear?

Have you ever seen pictures of your nursery or bedroom as a baby and young child? What colors were the walls painted? Did you have any gendered decorations? How did you feel in this space as a kid, and what role did it have in your identity as you grew up? If you could have been your own interior decorator, what would your childhood room have looked like?

# We Grow Up with Gender Roles

We know that our past shapes our future and that we are influenced by the people who raised us. Think back to when you were growing up and the gender roles your parents/guardians had in your family. In the space below, draw a "family tree" or diagram of family and adult role models. Next to each person's name describe the gender roles they modeled for you. Then, write about how you think these people influenced your ideas on gender identity.

Think of the toys you played with as a child. Which ones were your favorites? Were you given gendered toys to play with, such as trucks and dolls, or did you get to pick them out yourself?

Lots of children play dress-up, which allows them imaginative play and the opportunity to try out different roles. As a child, who did you want to play for dress-up? What kinds of outfits did you wear to play dress-up? Did you feel pressure to only wear certain dress-up clothes because of others' expectations?

# I Want to Be _____ When I Grow Up

Many children dream of what kind of work they'll do when they grow up. Unfortunately, many of us are taught that some jobs are very gendered (which is also often reinforced by media) and this can limit our dreams when they don't align with our assigned gender. For this exercise, make a list of all the jobs you wanted to have when you grew up.

........................................................................................

........................................................................................

........................................................................................

........................................................................................

........................................................................................

Now take a moment to imagine yourself doing each of these jobs today. Do they bring to mind particular gender identities or stereotypes? In the space below, draw or write about what comes to mind.

Going through puberty can be a confusing, emotional time for anyone. Because sometimes gender identity is not realized until puberty, when our bodies start to develop and change, this phase can feel especially challenging when you are exploring your gender identity. Did you feel any hesitation or negative feelings about starting puberty, or specific kinds of discomfort when puberty started?

The changes that start in our bodies during puberty can cause people to want to hide themselves. Sometimes people will start wearing clothes that conceal their bodies, or they will want to stay in their room—whether it's to hide their chest development or facial hair, or for a host of other reasons. These feelings are all often part of discovering your gender identity. Did you (or do you currently) feel like you wanted to hide some of your body during puberty? What did you want to hide?

When we are teenagers, we might be taught the gender norms of our household and try to fit into them. We may be so overwhelmed and scared by our feelings about our gender identity that we try really hard to perform our assigned roles on the gender binary. When you were an adolescent, did you ever find yourself trying hard or going overboard to present as your assigned gender? What steps did you take and how did they make you feel?

As a child, do you remember ever wishing your role in society was in a gender other than the one you were assigned at birth? What were some of the ways you questioned the stereotypical ways society wanted you to act?

# It's Time to Call Attendance

Think back to when you were in elementary or middle school. Remember at the beginning of the day, when the teacher would call attendance and say your name out loud? Sometimes people get certain feelings when they hear their name called out loud. Listen to your body and pay attention to your physical and emotional reactions. Reflect on the feelings you felt both physically and emotionally when you heard the teacher call your name during roll call. Now imagine: What if you could have heard a different name from your teacher during roll call? Was there a name you wanted the teacher to call you instead? Imagine the teacher calling you by that name and reflect on how you feel hearing the new name versus the old name.

Middle school is a time when many people find their own friend group and start navigating their gender identity. Did your gender identity feel comfortable, uncomfortable, or somewhere in the middle? How did you express your gender during this time? What changes started around middle school for you?

When we are growing up, we learn about various gender stereotypes. They can be subtle, like "girls don't ask guys on dates," or they can be overt, like "boys cannot learn ballet." Often, we are not even aware that we are learning these gender stereotypes, because they are so societally ingrained. Think back on when you grew up and write down some gender stereotypes you were taught.

Your gender identity can come from many different influences. Sometimes we see people in media or on television who have just the "look" we are going for. Did you ever see someone on television or in the media whose image you felt reflected who you really are? What were they wearing and how did they carry themselves that made you aspire to be like them?

## An Outfit of Your Dreams

When you were young, did your parents or guardians pick out your clothes for you to wear in the morning? Did you have any choice in the style or color of your clothes, or did your caregivers buy or obtain all your clothing? If you could go back in time and have complete control over your wardrobe, what would you have picked out in elementary school? In middle school? Visualize what your style or favorite outfit might have been in elementary, middle, and high school. Do you notice any differences between the outfits you were given and what you like? Imagine these younger versions of you in the outfits of your dreams. Do you feel any joy in imagining what your personal favorite outfits would be?

We know that people can make assumptions about our gender identity, and how others feel about us can affect how we feel about ourselves. Sometimes it's hard to separate how we feel about ourselves from how other people feel about us. How have people reacted to your gender expression in the past, both when you were following the gender norms of your assigned gender and when you were not?

Sometimes we have other people telling us how we can express our gender identity when we are kids and teenagers. Your parents might have made you wear a suit to prom, or you may have been told you couldn't cut your hair a certain way. When people tell us how we can and can't express ourselves, it can feel like we are boxed in. Did you feel in control or not in control of how you socially expressed your gender identity in the past? How so?

We know there are stereotypes about how men and women are "supposed" to act. You may have been told that people of your assigned gender were only allowed to do certain things or play in a certain way. Maybe you were told you couldn't go down a career path or pursue a certain goal because of gender stereotypes. What did you feel like when you realized these were just stereotypes? How did it feel to know you could break those stereotypes?

The way you currently present your gender identity may feel uncomfortable or make you feel uneasy. This could be a small, nagging feeling that has grown over many years, or your gender presentation could have just started to feel uncomfortable. Can you make any connections between how you felt about your gender identity when you were growing up and how you feel now?

_____

_____

_____

_____

_____

_____

_____

_____

_____

_____

_____

_____

_____

_____

# Birthday Reflections for the Past and Future

Sometimes birthdays are an opportunity to reflect on who we are and how we've changed over the years. Think back to several of your birthdays and try to remember the feelings you had related to your gender identity and presentation on those days. Write down five to ten words to describe the feelings you experienced on those days. Are these memories about your identity happy ones or do they make you uncomfortable? Now write down five to ten words you would like to feel about your gender identity on your birthday in three years.

You may have already been exploring your gender identity but have not quite put a name to the exploration. Sometimes people will start painting their nails clear or different colors, or they may progressively cut their hair shorter over time. When we do this, we may not consciously be aware that we are exploring different gender identities; we may just be looking for a change in life. Have you already done anything to change your outward expression that could be considered exploring your gender identity?

"THE WORLD MAKES YOU
SOMETHING YOU ARE NOT,
BUT YOU KNOW INSIDE
WHAT YOU ARE, AND
THAT QUESTION BURNS
IN YOUR HEART, HOW WILL
YOU BECOME THAT?"

— *GEENA ROCERO*

" WHO AM I? WHO AM I TO ME? . . .
HOW DO WE BETTER LISTEN
TO OURSELVES?
HOW DO WE STOP
SHUTTING OUT THE TRUTHS
THAT WE ARE AFRAID TO
RECOGNIZE AND START
SHUTTING OUT THE VOICES
THAT REBUT US? "

—*JANET MOCK*

# 3

# Discovering Who You Are

You have now done some of the hard work of facing your fears and the obstacles in the way of embracing your gender identity. You have also reflected on your childhood and the gender constructs that have been placed upon you. Now it's time to process those reflections and perhaps uncover some truths about yourself that those reflections may point to. It's also a good time to think about steps you may take to affirm your life and identity. In this section, you will actively explore your personal gender identity.

Our sense of self comes from all of our various identities wrapped into one. What are some identities you hold that are important to you, in addition to your gender identity? Are you a parent, a sibling, an aunt, uncle, or auncle? Are you an artist or athlete or entrepreneur? How does your ethnicity or background factor into your identity? What are some other aspects of what makes you uniquely *you*?

All of our identities have layers. Most of the younger layers of our identity come from the constructs that society and our families of origin place on us. If you hadn't had gender norms placed upon you in your younger years, do you believe you would have the same relationship to your gender identity as you do now? What do you think your gender expression would be without these influences? Can you describe it?

# An Excavation of Gender Identity

Imagine an archeologist has started an archeological dig of your gender identity over your lifetime. They are digging through your life layer by layer, each layer of the dig representing a year, or a few years, of your life. What would each layer represent in terms of your gender identity? Write down or draw what the team would find out about your gender identity from each layer of the dig.

How we wear our hair can play a significant role in how we express our gender identity. We are taught from a young age that girls have long hair and boys have short hair, though these norms are often broken. Do you feel like you need a different hairstyle or length in order to present as your gender identity? Why or why not?

Sometimes when you know, you know. Your gender identity can be something you just know. Stop to reflect and look inward and ask yourself, "Do I have a feeling that I just know what my gender identity is?" Even if you don't know everything for sure, are there any areas where you have certainty?

Think about the other roles you hold in your life, such as caretaker, friend, employee, or parent. When you think of yourself in these different roles, do you have a sense of your gender identity within them? How do you see yourself in relation to other people in your life? Is your role with them gendered?

When you are exploring your gender identity, it's important to look for clues about your feelings around gender norms and how you are presenting to the world. If you have uneasy feelings when you start to think about your own body, it may be time to seek help. Do you feel any discomfort when you think about yourself as your assigned gender? Can you describe that discomfort? Is investigating it an important part of your gender identity journey?

# Noticing the Norms

Sometimes we feel as if we must comply with all of society's norms to be successful. Take out a piece of paper and tear it into small pieces, writing down on each piece all of the stereotypical gender norms you feel like you are expected to live up to. The stereotypical norms include everything from hairstyles to opening doors for others to how vocal you are or are not at work. Now place them into two piles: one for norms that are comfortable to you and one for norms that feel uncomfortable. Look at the piles and see if you notice any patterns. Think about the emotions you experienced as you placed norms in the "uncomfortable" pile. Did you feel a sense of relief or sadness? Noticing norms can help bring awareness to the ways we feel pressured to comply with the gender binary and open possibility for relief and gentle acceptance, giving us space to realize: "No, that is not who I am."

It can be scary to admit to yourself that there is another gender presentation you'd feel more comfortable with. But this journal is a safe space, and these questions are only for you. If you have discomfort about your assigned gender, have you noticed that there's another gender you resonate with more? What about it resonates with you?

Just for today, imagine that you could wear whatever you wanted to work or school without fear of repercussions. What would you wear? What would your "look" be?

# A Picture of Me

Everyone has multiple identities. We have identities at work, at school, with friends, on social media, and in our own minds. Take some time to write down some of the identities you have held. Have you ever presented as more masculine, feminine, or androgynous with your friends? Does your gender expression change depending on who you're with or what situation you're in? Have you ever held a different identity on social media or in a video game? Keeping all of this in mind, imagine and draw your ideal avatar or profile picture of yourself. It can be human, animal, or a fantasy character from a video game—anything! When your imagination is limitless, what would a picture of you look like?

Does it ever feel like the gender identity you present to others is like wearing a costume? Do you feel like the clothes you wear and how you present yourself are just you playing a gendered role that you don't really align with? Write about how true or untrue this feels for you, and why you think that is.

Each year many people celebrate Mother's Day and Father's Day. What do these days mean for you and your gender identity? If you are or plan to be a parent, would you feel more comfortable celebrating Parents' Day? If you don't plan to be a parent, how would you like young children to see you? Would you want to be called a traditionally gendered name, or would you like something else more neutral?

# Standing Out in a Crowd

Actively exploring your gender identity is a process of mental and emotional exploration—and, at times, social exploration. Think of the last time you went to a party or family function. Many of us get nervous in large gatherings, but sometimes our nerves can be deeper than just social anxiety. Were you nervous at your last function due to the way you had to present yourself through your gender expression? Did you feel uneasy if you were presenting as your assigned gender, or were you comfortable? Take some time to reflect on your feelings from the last time you were in a large group or in front of several people at once. Imagine the next time you are in front of a several people or at a party. What would be your ideal gender expression? In the space below, draw or write about the "look" you would most like to have at your next big gathering.

Exploring your gender identity can result in wanting to make some changes to your current gender expression and presentation. These can be inward or outward changes. In private, when you mentally think of yourself, how do you want to express your gender identity? If there was no one to tell you otherwise, who would you be?

Hearing other people say our pronouns (for example, she/her/hers, he/him/his, they/them/theirs, ze/zir/zirs, etc.) is something a lot of people don't pay attention to. But if you are consistently being addressed by pronouns that do not align with your gender identity, it can be damaging to your mental health. How do you feel your current pronouns are, or are not, aligned with your gender identity? When other people refer to you with your pronouns, how does it make you feel?

Many trans and nonbinary people look in the mirror and want to see a flatter chest on their bodies. Have you ever thought about having a flatter chest? Would you ever consider buying a binder for your chest to feel more comfortable in yourself? Others look in the mirror and want to see a more developed chest, or feel discomfort if they have chest hair. If you have felt this way, would you ever consider wearing breast forms, taking hormones, or removing hair to better express your gender identity? When you think about your chest, what would you like it to look like or feel like?

# I Am _____

There are many terms we can use to name our gender identities. Go back to the terms section of this journal (see page ix) and explore whether any of the terms listed resonate with you. You can experiment by saying a sentence for each identity that begins with "I am [cisgender, agender, etc.]." Do any of these sentences feel more comfortable to you as you are saying them? Write down which sentences feel the most comfortable and uncomfortable.

| Comfortable | Uncomfortable |
| --- | --- |
| | |
| | |
| | |
| | |
| | |
| | |
| | |
| | |

Recognizing which descriptors feel most comfortable to you is vital because it allows you to know yourself better, and more easily share with others who you are. Now, imagine saying this comfortable sentence to another person and feel the emotions it brings up.

Now that you have taken time to actively explore your gender identity in this journal, do you feel like you have a new understanding of your gender identity? Is there anything that feels clearer? Is there anything that feels more confusing?

"HE ALLOWED HIMSELF
TO BE SWAYED BY HIS
CONVICTION THAT HUMAN
BEINGS ARE NOT BORN
ONCE...BUT THAT LIFE
OBLIGES THEM OVER AND
OVER AGAIN TO GIVE
BIRTH TO THEMSELVES."

—GABRIEL GARCÍA MÁRQUEZ

"I'M NOT WEARING A SKIN THAT I DON'T FEEL I AM ANYMORE. I'M NOT PLAYING A PERSONA; I'M NOT TRYING TO BE SOMETHING I'M NOT ANYMORE. I DON'T FEEL LIKE I'M STUCK IN THIS WEIRD MOMENT OF IN-BETWEEN."

—*NATHAN WESTLING*

# 4

# Building Your Support System

While you may think that exploring your gender identity is something you have to do alone, it does not have to be a lonely process. You can ask friends, family, or loved ones to join you in this exploration to show you support. You can also find support online. Yes, it can be nerve-racking to come out to people as gender questioning or gender nonconforming, but this section will help you plan to do so in a way that feels affirming, safe, and empowering for you.

We generally have a core group of friends and family who are closest to us. Think about some times you had to tell people something and you worried about their reaction. During these times, who are the people who offered you love and kindness? With whom in your core group would you feel most comfortable talking about your gender identity exploration and asking for support?

If you wanted to come out to someone, who would be the first person you would pick? Who feels like the safest friend or family member? Now that you have a person in mind, start to think about the words you would say to them. You can practice by writing what you would say on this page.

Everyone can feel lonely and isolated at times. Not only can it feel impossible to reach out for support, it can be hard to even pinpoint what kind of support we want or need. Think about how you would like to be supported when you're feeling alone. What would make you feel connected? For instance, do you like hugs, just knowing there are others like you around, or to talk things out?

If we can realize we need support *before* we get too depressed or anxious, it can help a lot. When have you found yourself wishing you had asked for help sooner? What are some cues that let you know you need the support of others?

Lots of people get anxious when thinking about coming out to their parents or parent figures, often because they may not share the same belief system. What about you? What emotions come to mind when you think about coming out to the people who raised you? If you are feeling anxious about coming out to them, what friend could you talk to about it?

# Long or Short Story

Explaining to someone that you're questioning your gender can be as simple as just saying that sentence. Or there may be people with whom you choose to elaborate about your deeper feelings. Close your eyes and imagine the first three to five people you want to tell that you're questioning your gender identity. For each person, imagine if you would prefer to give them a long or short explanation. Remember, it is up to you. You don't owe anyone your story, and it is yours to keep to yourself if you want to. In the space below, take a stab at writing out the short and long versions of the story you would share.

**The Short Story**

_____

_____

_____

**The Long Story**

_____

_____

_____

_____

_____

_____

Think about coming out to someone as transgender, gender questioning, gender-queer, gender nonconforming, nonbinary, or not cisgender. Some of these terms may feel more powerful, true, final, joyful, or scary than others. Which of these terms feels most comforting for you to say to someone else? Is there a term that feels safer than the others, and why? How comfortable are you with saying you identify with any of these terms at this moment?

Whether at an in-person gathering or over group text, video chat, or a phone call, the way our friends communicate with us and in our presence can have a strong impact on our sense of physical and emotional safety. Look back at your last group text or call to mind the last conversation you had with a group of friends. Do you remember your friends saying anything transphobic or homophobic? Does it feel like your friends are accepting of the trans and gender nonconforming community? When you reflect on past conversations with friends, do they feel like safe people to come out to? Why do they feel safe or unsafe?

The way in which we plan to come out to people can make a big difference in our comfort level and readiness. Some people may only be comfortable coming out through email or text and aren't ready for face-to-face yet. In which way would it feel safer for you to come out as questioning your gender identity—in person, by phone, or via text, email, or letter? Why does it feel safer?

# Compassion in a Letter

A powerful tool for overcoming fear and anxiety is to use mindful self-compassion to write a kind letter to yourself. Imagine you are writing a letter to a best friend who is questioning their gender and wants to come out to others. What compassionate things would you say to them to give them courage to come out? Use this space to write this letter and address it to yourself.

Are you active on social media? Some social media communities feel safe, while others may feel unsafe. Think about the social media communities you're a part of. Are there any that make you feel unsafe mentally and emotionally? If so, what are two coping skills you can use to protect yourself? What social media communities do you feel safest in, and why?

Coming out is a personal process that is unique to everyone, and for many people it involves varying degrees of coming out online. Some people may first come out with a new name or pronouns, while others may start with a different profile picture or gaming avatar. Is coming out on social media something you want to do? How would you feel safe doing so? Which of your social media communities would you feel safest coming out to? Are you interested in seeking out new online communities that are affirming and supportive for people exploring their gender identities?

# Are Your Online Communities Affirming?

There are many different opportunities to find a supportive online community. Social media platforms such as Facebook, Twitter, Reddit, Discord, Instagram, and TikTok all have different and unique qualities that allow people to be connected. Think about each social media platform you're on, take a look around recent conversations and posts, and see which groups or threads feel supportive and free from bullying, mocking, and attacks. Some questions you might ask yourself are:

- Do I feel comfortable fully expressing myself in this group?

- Are people subtly or overtly bullying others based on their gender identity or sexuality?

- Do people seem to gang up on each other?

- Are people reflective with each other when they disagree about something?

Look at each group or thread's privacy settings and reflect on how safe you feel in each community, either anonymously or not. Think about whether these communities are serving you, and give yourself permission to leave the ones where you don't feel safe or affirmed.

Do you feel like being in a room, either in person or virtually, with other people who are trans, gender nonconforming, or questioning their gender would be helpful for you? How would it be for you to hear other people's stories? Would you need a friend to come with you? Would it be helpful to call or text the group leader to get a feel for what the group is like first? What would make you most comfortable and ready to go to a support group meeting?

Let's say you have decided to come out to at least one person. It may be a friend, family member, or someone you met online. In what ways would you want this person to support you and support your gender identity? How can they help you? Would you feel comfortable telling them what kind of support you need from them?

"I THINK THAT A LOT OF
TIMES GENDER IS USED
TO SEPARATE AND DIVIDE.
IT'S THIS SOCIAL CONSTRUCT
THAT I DON'T REALLY FEEL
LIKE I FIT INTO THE WAY
I USED TO."

—*JONATHAN VAN NESS*

"... UNDERSTAND THAT WE ARE PEOPLE. WE'RE HUMAN BEINGS, AND THIS IS A HUMAN LIFE. THIS IS REALITY FOR US, AND ALL WE ASK FOR IS ACCEPTANCE AND WHAT WE SAY THAT WE ARE. IT'S A BASIC HUMAN RIGHT."

—ANDREJA PEJIC

# 5

# Handling Negativity

Exploring your gender identity can be difficult when so much anxiety, fear, and negativity are associated with questioning one's gender and being gender nonconforming. These emotions can come from other people, and they can come from within. In this section, you will begin to explore where these emotions come from, and you will learn tools to help you cope with negative feelings and to build your self-esteem.

It can be scary to come out to people who may not have been as supportive as you would have liked them to be in the past. Who are the important people in your life that you are most nervous or fearful to tell that you are questioning your gender identity? What kind of relationship have you had with them in the past, and how has that influenced your feelings about them now?

In what ways is your fear of what other people think of you controlling the narrative of your gender identity? Do you feel like your fear of what others think of you is pushing you to not accept your gender identity? Do you think this fear is holding you back from being yourself?

Shame is generally defined as the feeling a person has that something is wrong with them. Sometimes people can feel shameful about their gender identity because they think it is outside of the "norms" of society. Other people might feel shame because of how they were raised, or because of cultural or religious connections. Some people do not go through a period of shame at all. Do you have any shame about your gender identity? How does this shame block you from being your authentic self?

# Setting Boundaries Around Negativity

When you mention the LGBTQIA community to the people you interact with in your life, how do they react? Have they made negative comments about trans or gender nonconforming people in the past? Take some time to write down the name of anyone in your life who you feel might be transphobic or not accepting of diverse gender identities. Now write down the ways you are willing to deal with each of these people that would best honor and support yourself, such as having a heart-to-heart talk with them, giving them books or articles to read, setting some kind of boundary, or even deciding to cut them out of your life.

What parts of yourself are you proud of? If someone asked you about your greatest talents or qualities, what would they be? Try to be honest and introspective and really think about the positive. Even the slightest bit of positivity still counts. Reminding yourself of your positive qualities can give you an instant boost to your self-esteem when you are feeling down.

Most people struggle at times with feelings of low self-worth. It may feel hard to put into words the things you do well or to come up with positive words to write about yourself. Take a moment to try to step away from yourself and see yourself from other people's perspectives. What are the qualities that your partner, best friend, or someone else who loves you would say make you unique? Can you see these qualities in yourself?

What we see in society can affect our moods and outlook on life. If we see that the trans and gender nonconforming community is being treated poorly on a national or local level, it can have an effect on how we personally see the trans and gender nonconforming community—and ourselves within it. What do you see about how trans and gender nonconforming people are treated in society or your community that affects you, either negatively or positively?

# Put Yourself in the Chair

During moments when you experience gender dysphoria or transphobia, it's important to extend compassion towards yourself. This exercise, adapted from the empty chair technique in Gestalt therapy, will help you do that. Gestalt therapy focuses on the present and often uses role playing to gain awareness of your present and to make positive change.

To start, place two chairs facing each other. Sit down in one of the chairs and imagine yourself sitting in the other chair. When you look at your other self, try to be as compassionate as possible. Start talking to your "self" in the other chair and telling them all the positive qualities they/you possess. Practice telling that other you what you know to be their strengths and values. Complete the exercise by looking at yourself in the other chair and telling them "I love you."

Do you see transphobia in the media that you consume? Do you read the news and see anti-trans legislation being proposed or passing in your community? Sometimes transphobia occurs in subtle microaggressions that not everyone notices, and all of these negative messages can be incredibly painful. How do you think this negativity affects your sense of the worthiness of trans and gender non-conforming people, and comfort with exploring your own gender identity?

If you experience shame about your gender identity, what are some coping skills you can use when you feel like you are getting into a shame spiral? Write down at least three things you can do to take care of yourself, such as alternative activities or positive sayings you can repeat to yourself.

# Shame Is Not Your Fault

Earlier in this journal, you read about how the messaging we received in childhood can affect our construct of gender. This, along with the media we consume, can lead to feelings of shame about our gender identity. Think back to the last time you felt shame about your gender identity. Now try to imagine the source of this shame. Was it rooted in the past, or was it caused by something you felt or saw recently? How do you feel like you have been taught to feel shame about your gender identity? If someone or something else has taught you to feel this shame, try writing an apology to yourself from the perspective of that person or thing.

Do you find yourself putting off your gender exploration because you feel guilty about how your gender identity will affect other people? Maybe you are worried that a parent or spouse will be upset that their child or partner is transgender, and you don't want to hurt them. Imagine if this guilt were lifted—how far along would you be in your gender exploration now? If you're not dealing with feelings of guilt, what are some other emotions you have about how your gender identity might impact others?

Do you feel anxious that friends or family members will mock or discourage you if you tell them you are exploring your gender? Or perhaps you are afraid of how people will react when you are moving down the street. Know that these fears may be valid and try to treat them with tenderness. Can you think of a time in your life when you put aside fear of what other people thought and did something anyway? How did that feel?

Many people who are exploring their gender identity or are transgender have never met another transgender person. Being part of a queer community can help you feel safe, supported, and connected. What transgender and queer figures do you know and admire? Are there qualities they possess that you might have, too? Is there anyone, in person or online, to whom you would like to reach out to build community?

Transphobia or fear about transitioning could have been instilled in you at a young age through the messaging you received from your family, community, culture, or religion. If you feel fear of coming out or if you have negative feelings about trans and gender nonconforming people, when do you think these feelings and emotions first started? Where in your life do you think they came from?

Research shows that resiliency—the ability to bounce back or recover from challenges or setbacks—can be a protective factor against internalized transphobia or shame about questioning your gender identity. When you think of yourself as being resilient, what qualities of yours come to mind? When you have been faced with adversity, either in the past or more recently, what qualities do you have that helped you overcome a challenge or problem?

# "Hear Me Roar"

Sometimes we are strong and don't even realize it. It takes a purposeful inward eye to realize all the moments we have shown emotional strength. Being strong can be anything from saying no to harmful people or behaviors, to letting yourself cry, to asking for help when you need it. Write three to five sentences that begin with "I am strong when I . . ."

Anxiety can come in the form of fear, worry, or panic. It can be helpful to have a plan—or a toolbox of coping skills—for dealing with the emotions before they arrive so that you can be ready to deal with them when they come. What are some things you can do to take care of yourself when you feel anxiety starting to creep up (such as taking deep breaths or going for a walk)? What kind of plan can you create with these tools?

People say that laughter is medicine, and it really is! Laughing lets you release your emotions and sends you into a state of relaxation. It lowers your blood pressure and initiates the release of those feel-good chemicals your body needs. What makes you laugh? What are some ways you can bring more laughter into your life?

"IF I WAIT FOR
SOMEONE ELSE
TO VALIDATE MY
EXISTENCE, IT WILL
MEAN THAT I'M
SHORTCHANGING
MYSELF."

—*ZANELE MUHOLI*

WE EACH HAVE TO
FIND OUR OWN COPING
MECHANISMS—AND THIS
ISN'T JUST IN TERMS OF
THE HESITATION OF FINDING
OUR VOICE, BUT IN
HOW WE DEAL WITH
OUR OWN STRESS.

—*MICHELLE OBAMA*

# 6

# Practicing Self-Care

In this journal, you have recognized how important a support system is during your gender exploration and have named some ways you can find support. Now is the time to reflect on your own self-care. You are embarking on an important journey, and it is important to stay mentally and emotionally healthy throughout. The most important tools for maintaining this health are practicing self-care and self-acceptance and learning to have self-love.

# Self-Care Quiz

*Let's start off with a quiz about your current self-care practices:*

Do you get enough sleep?  **Y / N**

Do you eat meals regularly and give your body nourishment every day?  **Y / N**

Do you meditate or practice mindfulness?  **Y / N**

Do you take the time to nourish your mind by reading, practicing a hobby, or learning new things?  **Y / N**

Do you consistently take care of daily living activities like taking showers, brushing your hair, and brushing your teeth?  **Y / N**

Do you exercise or at least spend some time outside every day?  **Y / N**

[
- If you answered mostly yeses, you likely have strong systems in place to provide yourself self-care.

- If you answered mostly noes, you may find that focusing on adding more self-care into your life will help improve your mental and physical health.
]

What ways do you currently practice self-care and how often do you practice these things?

-------------------------------------------------------------------

-------------------------------------------------------------------

-------------------------------------------------------------------

-------------------------------------------------------------------

-------------------------------------------------------------------

Lots of people think of self-care and imagine something like relaxing in a bath-tub or getting a massage. While those things can be soothing, consistent, daily self-care is often simpler. What does self-care mean to you? What are some cues that tell you that you are practicing self-care?

We all experience times in our lives when we are unkind to ourselves. Sometimes we may say mean things or judge ourselves harshly. If you find that your internal dialogue is filled with negative statements about yourself, try replacing those statements with kind words instead. What are three to five kind statements you can say to yourself throughout this week?

Gender euphoria is when you feel a sense of happiness over something to do with your gender presentation, body, gender identity, or how others treat you. It can feel amazing, but there can sometimes be low periods of dysphoria afterward. If you have a low period like this, how would you take care of yourself? What would your first go-to coping skill be? What would calm you down and ground you? Write down three self-care routines that would help.

You can have so much hustle and bustle in your life that you forget to prioritize your self-care. Have there been times in the past when you were so busy you forgot to take care of yourself? What happened?

What are some signs that you need to slow down and make time for yourself? These signs could be physical, emotional, behavioral, or anything else that says "Take care of me!"

_____

_____

_____

_____

_____

_____

_____

_____

_____

_____

_____

_____

_____

_____

_____

# Soothe Yourself

Sometimes, when we get very anxious or are having a difficult emotion, it can help to stop and ground ourselves and practice mindfulness and self-compassion. A way to self-soothe during a difficult emotion is to cradle your chin in your hand and just feel the warmth of your hand on your chin. If your chin causes you to feel dysphoria, there are other places you could cradle, such as putting a hand on one of your knees or holding your calf. If you feel comfortable doing so, you could place your hand over your heart or give yourself a hug. Take some time to practice this gentle kindness and calmly hold yourself like you love yourself. Other self-soothing activities you might engage in include:

- Cuddling with a stuffed animal or soft toy

- Smelling satchels that are filled with scents like lavender and chamomile.

- Doing something with your hands, such as playing with a fidget toy.

- Exercising your creative side by drawing or painting.

Sometimes we think we are giving ourselves self-care, but it might not be in the healthiest of ways (such as turning to substances or behaviors that cause us to numb out or avoid our feelings, or engaging in actions harmful to ourselves or others). What are some of the healthiest ways that you practice self-care now? Are there any forms of self-care you have wanted to try before but haven't yet?

So far in this journal, you have taken a very personal, introspective look at yourself and your gender identity. You may have found answers you didn't know were there, or you may have allowed buried feelings to come to the surface. How are you feeling after working through this gender exploration journal so far? Are there ways you are feeling uncomfortable? Are there ways you are feeling more at ease?

Are there things you do to comfort yourself that are unhealthy? Or are there important self-care routines that you have a hard time accomplishing? How can you turn these habits into acts of care and kindness to yourself? Write at least two unhealthy habits and your plans to change them to healthier habits.

Sometimes we just keep going through life on our own and don't realize when our emotions have gotten to the point where we need extra help. If you stop to think and reflect, do you feel like you have had periods of depression, anxiety, or thoughts of hurting yourself? Do you have any past trauma that you have not yet explored in a safe, professional environment? If you have any of these feelings, or feel so overwhelmed that it's hard to do the things you need to do in life, it's probably time to seek the help of a mental health professional. In the Resources section (page 148), there is information on directories that you can use to search for a therapist in your area. Do you feel like seeing a counselor or therapist would be beneficial to you? Would you be willing to seek help?

# Celebrate Your Milestones with Joy

It has been said that patience is a virtue. In many ways, patience can be helpful for reducing anxiety and allowing us to wait when needed. Sometimes we don't get what we need immediately, and especially with a transition, those needs can take some time. No matter where you are in your journey, the passage of time can be frustrating. Take a moment to write down ways you will have patience and celebrate who you are along the way. For instance, are there holidays or special occasions you will be looking forward to, even while you're in the process of affirming yourself? Are there any milestones that you want to celebrate?

Sometimes just talking or writing about feelings, whether positive or negative, can be overwhelming. Using this journal may have been overwhelming for you at times. Processing feelings and emotions through journaling can be empowering and exciting, but it can also be exhausting and require us to be a little extra gentle with ourselves. What are some ways you will practice self-care after you use this journal?

Our greatest cheerleaders are often ourselves, especially at times when we feel we have no one else in our corner. When was the last time you were your own cheerleader? In what ways can you cheer yourself on during this process of introspection, discovery, and gender exploration?

You have embarked on a journey of self-reflection in this journal to explore your gender identity. In doing so, it's possible that you may become impatient to start exploring your gender identity further. If this sense of impatience occurs, what are some things you could tell yourself to put your feelings into perspective? In the past, how have you used self-care to calm impatience?

"BELIEVE IN YOURSELF. YOU'VE GOT TO TAKE THAT CHANCE, EVEN IF IT'S HARD, EVEN IF IT DOESN'T MAKE SENSE: JUST BELIEVE IN YOURSELF. EVEN IF YOU DON'T, PRETEND THAT YOU DO AND, AT SOME POINT, YOU WILL. WITH SELF-BELIEF COMES SELF-ESTEEM."

—VENUS WILLIAMS

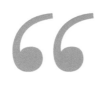 I HAVE LEARNED
OVER THE YEARS
THAT WHEN ONE'S
MIND IS MADE UP, THIS
DIMINISHES FEAR;
KNOWING WHAT MUST
BE DONE DOES AWAY
WITH FEAR.

—*ROSA PARKS*

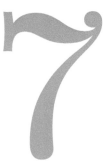

# Embracing Your
# Gender Identity

Now that you have explored your gender identity in the last six sections of your journal, you may be wondering what your next steps will be. This section will help you explore ways to express your gender, come out to others, and make peace with the gender identity that you have discovered. If you have questions about how to integrate your gender identity into your life, this section can help you.

You have now undergone a deep, reflective exploration of your gender identity and how it relates to yourself and other aspects of your life. While you may not know yet exactly how you want to define yourself or if you need to transition, you may have a clearer understanding of what your gender identity is. What conclusions have you come to about your gender identity after working through this journal?

_____

_____

_____

_____

_____

_____

_____

_____

_____

_____

_____

_____

_____

Some people feel like they would be more comfortable if they made physical changes that aligned with their gender. What changes, if any, would you consider making?

_____

_____

_____

_____

_____

_____

_____

_____

_____

_____

_____

_____

_____

_____

_____

While it's possible that you have come to some strong conclusions about your gender identity, you may still have many questions you need answered before you fully embrace your gender identity. Do you feel like you still have some uncertainty about your gender identity? How so?

_____

_____

_____

_____

_____

_____

_____

_____

_____

_____

_____

_____

_____

_____

Having some uncertainty about your gender identity is perfectly normal, even after so much processing. Sometimes finding your gender identity just takes more time. Even people who have transitioned may continue to feel uncertainty about their identities. This is, again, normal, and you're not alone. Even if you don't have complete certainty about your gender identity, you can still feel confident about other aspects of your life. Can you write down ways you can feel confident even through uncertainty, such as knowing what your positive qualities are?

# The Roles We Play Every Day

Think about your daily schedule and the people you regularly encounter. What roles do you play throughout the week? Maybe you are a student, manager, child, parent, or spouse. In each of these roles, how do you currently express your gender identity? Write about each of your roles and ask yourself if you would rather express your gender differently in these roles. Would you be willing to express your gender identity like this every day?

Exploring your gender can lead to acceptance of your identity and a strong willingness to change. It can also lead to even more questions and uncertainty than you had in the beginning. How do you feel now that you have explored your gender identity? Do you feel acceptance, or do you feel fear and hesitation? If you feel fear or hesitation, I encourage you to reach out to your support system.

You don't have to have all of the answers about your gender identity right now. Knowing yourself is a lifelong project, and that includes knowing your gender identity. What's important is to accept where you are in this present moment with openness and compassion. In this moment, right now, what do you know about your gender identity?

Now that you've explored your gender identity, you might want to start living differently. Do you want to change or transition something about your gender expression and presentation? What are some ways you might want to do this?

_____

_____

_____

_____

_____

_____

_____

_____

_____

_____

_____

_____

_____

_____

## What If There Was a Miracle?

In solution-focused brief therapy, there's something called the miracle question, which can help us more clearly know what we want. If there was a miracle today that allowed you to express yourself in any way you wanted to, how would you express your gender? This miracle would take away any naysayers about your gender identity, and you could fully express yourself as you are without any fear. Who would you be and how would you present in public? Draw or write about your "miracle self" in the space below.

The exploration you've made in this journal may have brought up some big emotions. You may have felt upset with yourself along the way or experienced feelings of self-doubt or shame. Now—and always—is a great time to practice self-care to show yourself some love and encouragement. What are some ways you can wrap yourself in love and take care of yourself?

Sometimes it can be hard to hear our inner voice in the midst of all the other noise inside our heads. What do you hear when you listen to your inner voice? What are some ways you can tell the difference between your own voice and the other messages and voices in life that are trying to get your attention?

There's a lot to think about with gender transition. You may have started to think about the logistics of coming out to other people in your life, and it may feel daunting. How do you think your family, friends, and colleagues would respond to your coming out? Do you think you can be happy and at peace with yourself even if their response is not what you had hoped for?

# Nurturing a Calm Connection to Yourself

By using this journal and completing the prompts and exercises, you may have dealt with fears, worries, disagreements within yourself, or feelings of sadness at times. You may have also been happy, excited, joyful, or felt a sense of calm. No matter how you felt, it took courage to journal your thoughts and feelings about your gender identity. When you have just experienced an emotional journey, it can be helpful to stop and reconnect with yourself. Try to write three kind and compassionate sentences to yourself that would help give you a sense of calm.

1. .......................................................................................................................

.......................................................................................................................

.......................................................................................................................

2. .......................................................................................................................

.......................................................................................................................

.......................................................................................................................

3. .......................................................................................................................

.......................................................................................................................

.......................................................................................................................

If you decide to transition in order to affirm who you are, what would you need to change *inwardly*? Do you feel like you would need to work on any internalized transphobia, dysphoria, or insecurities? What are some ways you want to work on becoming more confident in your gender identity?

If you decide to transition, what would you need to change *outwardly*? Would you need a new wardrobe? When you think about how you are perceived by the world, are there parts of you that you want people to see differently, like your haircut or style?

# The Safest Person to Come Out To

Close your eyes and imagine it is time to come out to someone. Who would be the first person you would feel safe coming out to? There are lots of ways people come out to others, including through text, in person, or with a letter. When you imagine coming out to this safest person, how do you think you would come out to them? Now, imagine the words you would want to say or write. Would you feel safe and confident to come out to this person? Do you feel like you can come out to them in real life? Would you like to make a plan to do so?

If you encounter someone who is unkind to you about your gender identity, what is your plan to take care of your emotions? Write down some things you can do in the moment to remind yourself of your confidence and worth.

We all have internal resources to protect and support ourselves when people are being mean or causing us harm. This may be a voice in your head that gives you a pep talk, or it could be the ability to let what others say roll off your back. What internal protective factors do you have to support yourself when someone is unkind to you about your gender identity?

This journal has offered a path inward so that you might find some answers and peace as you explore your gender identity. After all that you have explored within yourself, and after looking at the support system you have, do you feel like transitioning is the next step in your life right now? If so, what is the first thing you would like to do?

"YOU LOOK RIDICULOUS
IF YOU DANCE,
YOU LOOK RIDICULOUS
IF YOU DON'T DANCE,
SO YOU MIGHT AS WELL
DANCE."

—*GERTRUDE STEIN*

# A FINAL WORD

You have just undertaken a great and in-depth exploration that let you reflect on your own gender identity. It took courage and the willingness to be introspective and honest. Now that you have reflected about your gender identity, you may feel more confident in expressing yourself as who you are. You may also still have questions. Know that wherever you are in your exploration is okay, and there is no "right" way to do this. Your exploration is as unique as you are.

I have worked with hundreds of people who have taken this journey to explore and come out as transgender, genderqueer, gender nonconforming, agender, nonbinary, and more. Many people have come back to see me again after transitioning, grateful to be living out the authentic expression of themselves and excited and with a spark back in their lives. This is not to say there will not be challenges in your life if you transition or change the way you express your gender. There might be that one family member who will never accept you, you may have to deal with microaggressions through-out your life, and there is the very real danger of transphobic harassment and being stymied by oppressive laws. But know that you are not alone and that there are communities ready to welcome you with open arms. There are supports out there for you, whether online or in person. This is only the beginning of living your life authentically, and I wish you the very best, wherever you are and wherever you choose to go.

# RESOURCES

**Trans Lifeline**—This is the only national hotline run by and for the trans community, offering peer support, microgrants, and more to trans people in crisis. 877-565-8860, TransLifeline.org

**The Trevor Project**—This is a crisis line for the LGBTQIA community that handles over 100,000 calls, chats, and texts every year through its website. TheTrevorProject.org

## BOOKS

*The Queer and Transgender Resilience Workbook: Skills for Navigating Sexual Orientation and Gender Expression,* by Anneliese Singh (New Harbinger Publications, 2018)

*The Reflective Workbook for Partners of Transgender People: Your Transition as Your Partner Transitions,* by D. M. Maynard (Jessica Kingsley Publishers, 2019)

*Sorted: Growing Up, Coming Out, and Finding My Place (A Transgender Memoir),* by Jackson Bird (Tiller Press, 2019)

*Trans Bodies, Trans Selves: A Resource for the Transgender Community,* edited by Laura Erickson-Schroth (Oxford University Press, 2014)

## ORGANIZATIONS

**Fenway Health**—Located in Boston, this is one of the nation's leading gender clinics, and it has medical resources as well as virtual support groups. FenwayHealth.org/care/medical/transgender-health

**PFLAG**—Both an advocacy organization and a network of support groups for the LGBTQIA community in all 50 states. PFLAG.org

**The Philadelphia Trans Wellness Conference**—A yearly supportive gathering for the transgender community as well as professionals. The community track is tailored to the trans community itself. MazzoniCenter.org

**Trevor Space**—This is the social arm of The Trevor Project, offering forums and conversations for people aged 13 to 24. TrevorSpace.org

## WEBSITES

**The National Center for Transgender Equality**—An excellent resource for learning about your rights. TransEquality.org

**TherapyDen**—A national database of therapists who care about social justice. You can search the site for a professional near you who matches your needs. TherapyDen.com

**Trans Student Educational Resources (TSER)**—This is a national, youth-led organization that empowers and advocates for trans and gender-nonconforming students. They offer training, information, and a scholarship program for trans students. TransStudent.org

**World Professional Association of Transgender Health**—Publishes the standards of care for working with transgender people in a healthcare setting. WPATH.org

**Finding an in-person or online support group:** If your area has a local LGBTQIA center, you can start there by checking their schedule of group meetings. You can also go to PFLAG.org and look up your local chapter. The Psychology Today website lets you search for support and therapy groups near you. Often, resources like Fenway Health offer online support groups. Another way to find a support group is to call a local gender-affirming therapist and ask them if they have a list to share with you. Trans Lifeline is also a good resource.

**Finding an affirming and supportive therapist or counselor:** There are several websites where you can search for therapists near you, including TherapyDen .com and PsychologyToday.com. Once there, you can filter by the terms "gender identity" or "transgender" to narrow your search. Look for therapists who speak about the transgender community or gender identity in their "About Me" section and have their pronouns listed on their profile. When you call or email a therapist, ask them about their experience working with the transgender community and how they see themselves as affirming. They should be willing to speak openly about this, and you should feel comfortable with their answers. Another great way to find an affirming therapist is to ask someone in the transgender community for a recommendation or ask around at a trans support group you may attend.

# Acknowledgments

I would like to thank my clients for trusting me with their mental health care and allowing me to be part of their journeys.

Thank you, Joe, for the endless support, inspiration, and uplifting conversations, and for supporting my many endeavors.

Thank you, Mom and Jimmie, for being unconditionally supportive.

# About the Author

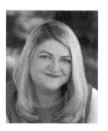

Katie Leikam, MBA, LCSW, is a gender therapist and small business owner with over 10 years of experience working with the LGBTQIA community. She is WPATH GEI SOC v7 certified. Katie serves the LGBTQIA, transgender, and genderqueer communities by working with her clients regarding gender identity, anxiety, autism, relationship stress, family and religious trauma, and coming out. Katie is also a speaker and educator, having spoken at conferences including Gender Odyssey Los Angeles and the United States Professional Association of Transgender Health. She offers consultation to other professionals.

Katie provides continuing education on the topics of gender identity and the LGBTQIA community, both in-person and via her online courses at the Clinician's LGBTQIA Learning Platform. She been quoted in many national publications as an expert in her field.